Abbas Hamieh

Challenges in Role Transition of New Nurse Graduates

AF135941

Abbas Hamieh

Challenges in Role Transition of New Nurse Graduates

LAP LAMBERT Academic Publishing

Impressum / Imprint

Bibliografische Information der Deutschen Nationalbibliothek: Die Deutsche Nationalbibliothek verzeichnet diese Publikation in der Deutschen Nationalbibliografie; detaillierte bibliografische Daten sind im Internet über http://dnb.d-nb.de abrufbar.
Alle in diesem Buch genannten Marken und Produktnamen unterliegen warenzeichen-, marken- oder patentrechtlichem Schutz bzw. sind Warenzeichen oder eingetragene Warenzeichen der jeweiligen Inhaber. Die Wiedergabe von Marken, Produktnamen, Gebrauchsnamen, Handelsnamen, Warenbezeichnungen u.s.w. in diesem Werk berechtigt auch ohne besondere Kennzeichnung nicht zu der Annahme, dass solche Namen im Sinne der Warenzeichen- und Markenschutzgesetzgebung als frei zu betrachten wären und daher von jedermann benutzt werden dürften.

Bibliographic information published by the Deutsche Nationalbibliothek: The Deutsche Nationalbibliothek lists this publication in the Deutsche Nationalbibliografie; detailed bibliographic data are available in the Internet at http://dnb.d-nb.de.
Any brand names and product names mentioned in this book are subject to trademark, brand or patent protection and are trademarks or registered trademarks of their respective holders. The use of brand names, product names, common names, trade names, product descriptions etc. even without a particular marking in this work is in no way to be construed to mean that such names may be regarded as unrestricted in respect of trademark and brand protection legislation and could thus be used by anyone.

Coverbild / Cover image: www.ingimage.com

Verlag / Publisher:
LAP LAMBERT Academic Publishing
ist ein Imprint der / is a trademark of
OmniScriptum GmbH & Co. KG
Heinrich-Böcking-Str. 6-8, 66121 Saarbrücken, Deutschland / Germany
Email: info@lap-publishing.com

Herstellung: siehe letzte Seite /
Printed at: see last page
ISBN: 978-3-659-62105-5

Copyright © 2014 OmniScriptum GmbH & Co. KG
Alle Rechte vorbehalten. / All rights reserved. Saarbrücken 2014

TABLE OF CONTENTS

APPENDICES

LIST OF TABLES

CHAPTER I

INTRODUCTION

A. Background

The nursing profession has gone through fundamental and evolutionary changes in the past decades in order to meet the demands of the growing complexities of the healthcare systems. The nursing shortage, one major stumbling block debilitating the nursing profession, has been well addressed locally and internationally over the past decade. The shortage of registered nurses (RNs) in the United States of America (USA) is estimated to reach 20% by year 2015(National Center for Health Workforce Analysis, 2002), while in Canada, it is estimated to reach 60,000 RNs by year 2022 (Canadian Nurse Association, 2007). In the "oil rich" Arabic speaking countries, El-Jardali et al. (2013) reported severe shortage of "internally trained nurses," while in Lebanon, few research studies indicated that the high turnover rate of RNs, ranging from 67.1% to 78.9% (El-Jardali et al., 2009a,b), and the high external migration rate of experienced nurses (El-Jardali et al., 2012), might have contributed to the shortage of RNs in difficult to staff areas (El-Jardali, et al., 2013).

Many recent research studies indicated that one of the sources contributing to the shortage of nursing professionals is the attrition of new graduate nurses (NGN/s) (Clark & Springer, 2012; Fielden, 2012; Holland & Moddeman, 2012; Kantar, 2012; Kramer, Maguire, Halfer, Brewer, & Schmalenberg, 2013). Kovenor, et al. (2007) reported that 13% of NGNs in USA changed their principal jobs after one year of practice and 37% intend to change their jobs in the near future. On the other hand, NGNs turnover rate in USA is reported at 35-60% (Institute of Medicine, 2005) and may reach 75% sometimes (Nursing Executive Center, 2005). In Canada, the NGN's

3

attrition rate is equal to 28% (Canadian Nurse Association, 2007), while in Lebanon, One in five University-prepared nurses migrate externally in the first two years after their graduation (El-Jardali, et al., 2008). In KSA, Fielden (2012) suggested that the more acceptance of nursing as a profession for both males and females, and the "Saudization policy" which ensued an expansion of local and international educational opportunities for Saudis are accountable for the increased number of NGNs entering the workforce.

The recent research studies also indicated that the high attrition rate of NGNs is related to many factors comparable to NGN's work environment (Clark & Springer, 2012; Fielden, 2012; Holland & Moddeman, 2012; Kantar, 2012; Kramer, Maguire, Halfer, Brewer, & Schmalenberg, 2013). Stress which is reported as a prevalent characteristic of the new graduate nurses' work environment (Bratt & Felzer, 2011; Kantar, 2012), occurs most severely during the role transition phase early in their practice (Kramer, Maguire, Brewer, & Schmalenberg, 2013). Furthermore, the build-up of stress levels may lead to anxiety (Kantar, 2012) which is manifested at manageable levels among NGNs (Washington, 2012). NGNs' Professional satisfaction, which is another factor contributing to NGNs' attrition, is related to the reality shock that new graduate nurses encounter during their transition into practice (Holland & Moddeman, 2012; Kramer, Brewer, & Maguire, 2013). Stress, anxiety, reality shock and professional satisfaction constitute a breadth of published research evidence addressing transition of new graduate nurses into practice.

The other breadth of research evidence addressing NGNs role transition is the evidence-based transition programs aimed at facilitating the transition experiences of NGNs. In the past three years, abundant research evidence had been published in this regard in support for the value of the transition programs in improving transition experiences of NGNs and their retention rates (Bratt & Felzer, 2011; Dyess & Parker, 2012; Fielden, 2012; Goode, Lynn, McElroy, Bednash, & Murray, 2013; Kowalski &

Cross, 2010; Kramer et al., 2012; Kramer, Maguire, Brewer, & Schmalenberg, 2013; Maxwell, 2011).

Goode, Lynn, McElroy, Bednash, & Murray (2013) recommended national accreditation of transition programs targeting NGNs. The authors argued that it is necessary to have national accreditation similar to other healthcare professions like medicine and pharmacy. The duration of the program is of high value in achieving the pronounced goals (Bratt & Felzer, 2011; Goode et al., 2013) and should be extended to one year (Goode et al., 2013) but not less than 6 months (Bratt & Felzer, 2011).

B. Significance

An initial electronic search for research literature addressing NGNs' role transition and published in the past three years, showed a scarcity of publications in the Arabic speaking countries compared to a plethora of publications in the non-Arabic speaking countries specifically in the USA, Australia, UK and Canada. This finding is consistent with the literature (Kantar, 2012; Rush, Adamack, Gordon, Lilly & Janke, 2013). In the light of the current nursing shortage in Lebanon (El-Jardali et al., 2007) which is potentiated by the high migration rate of University prepared Lebanese nurses (El-Jardali et al., 2012, El-Jardali et al., 2008), and in light of the nursing shortage in the middle east (El-Jardali, 2007), it is imperative to evaluate the NGN transition experiences in the middle-east as compared to the current literature in the developed countries.

Knowing that there is no comparative literature review that addressed this subject in the past three years, this review will provide valuable and current information about the subject. By understanding the challenges in role transition of NGNs, and by learning about its most reliable and valid measurement tools, nurse leaders and healthcare policy makers will be able to design the most convenient transition programs necessary to facilitate NGNs role transition in a middle-eastern context. This comparative literature review aims at exploring the transition challenges that new graduate nurses' encounter in the middle-east compared to USA.

CHAPTER II

METHOD

A. Stages of Integrative Research Review

1. *Formulation of the Problem*

- Search one

The first professional practice experience of new graduate nurses, in the Arabic speaking countries compared to other countries, is the ultimate subject of interest in this literature review. However, the literature encompasses an extensive number of publications of varied purposes and designs addressing this wide subject. An initial search for articles or reviews, in Scopus e-database, using the Boolean phrase (novice PRE/1 nurse*) OR (new* PRE/2 nurse*) OR (graduat* PRE/1 nurse*), and limited to the period between January 2010 and April 2013 returned 1575 articles. The search was further limited to articles written in English Language and addressing the subject of interest in USA, Australia, UK, New Zealand, Canada, Ireland and in the Arabic speaking countries. The number of articles was reduced to 661 articles. The list of key words that appeared with those 661 articles was also an extensive list. At this point it became imperative that the literature review should be narrowed down to specific variables of interest. Job satisfaction, one of the most interesting key words listed, appeared in 43 articles out of 661 articles.

The same search process was administered again in the e-databases CINAHL and PubMed. However, the search terms and Boolean phrases were altered as applicable to the search engines specified. Also, some limitations which are search engine-specific were applied in order to eliminate non-related articles. The result rendered was 13 articles from CINAHL and 18 articles from PubMed.

After completing this search, all citations (74 citations) from the three e-databases were uploaded to Refworks, an internet-based citation management software, and the list was further reduced to 59 citations by removing duplicates. Of these 59 articles, none was found to be related to the Arabic speaking countries. Therefore, a comparison between Arabic speaking countries and the rest of the world in regard to job satisfaction among new graduate nurses was not possible.

- Search two

In order to capture relevant published literature in the Arabic speaking countries and make a comparison with other countries, the same steps used in search one in the three e-databases were followed in search two with the key word "transition" instead of "job satisfaction." The result of search two, after removing all duplicates, was 136 articles. Then, the titles of all the articles were reviewed and the articles that do not address transition experiences of new graduate nurses were removed. This step further reduced the number of articles to 103 articles. At the end of this search process, many abstracts of the remaining 103 articles were reviewed and lead to the conclusion that the subject should be further narrowed down in order to capture articles with specific research purposes.

- Search three

The same search process of "search two" was followed in "search three" except that the Boolean phrases in the three e-databases were expanded to include the key word "challenge*." The purpose of this search was to capture published articles addressing "transition" and "challenge/s" and "new graduate nurses" at the same time. The result of this search rendered 30 articles. After removal of duplicate articles and review of the articles' titles, the result went down to 18 articles addressing transition challenges among new graduate nurses.

- Conclusion of search one, two and three

The three searches explained above have conveyed an overview of the available research literature addressing the main subject of interest within the past three years. The searches provided a synopsis of the key words that can be used to identify new graduate nurses and the challenges they face during their transition into professional practice. The searches also returned a large number of articles addressing the "nurse residency programs, the most widely spread strategy used by nurse leaders in an attempt to facilitate the transition of new graduate nurses into professional practice. Therefore, based on an overview of the available research literature in the past three years, the main subject of interest was narrowed down to two research questions:

1.   What are the challenges that the new graduate nurses (NGNs) face in the Arabic speaking countries compared to USA?

2.   What is/ are the most frequent, valid and reliable quantitative research instruments that measure the transition experiences of NGNs in the Arabic speaking countries and/ or USA?

2. Data Collection

New graduate nurses were variably identified in the literature as novice nurses, novice registered nurses, newly licensed registered nurses, newly licensed graduate nurses, newly licensed nurses, newly graduated registered nurses, newly graduating registered nurses, new nurses, new graduate nurses and new graduate registered nurses. This variability in the utilization of the defining keywords that resemble new graduate nurses is echoed in other literature reviews (Rush, Adamack, Gordon, Lilly and Janke , 2013). Therefore, in order to capture all research literature addressing new graduate nurses, the various NGN terminologies were used in the search fields of the three e-databases mentioned previously.

In Scopus, the Boolean phrase in the search field was defined as follows: ((novice PRE/1 nurse*) OR (new* PRE/2 nurse*) OR (graduat* PRE/1 nurse*)) AND (transition) AND (program* OR challenge*). The key word "New*" with the wildcard (*) are used to represent the words new or newly, while the key word "nurse*" represents the words nurse or nurses. The key word "graduat*" resembles the words graduate, graduating or graduated while the word "challenge*" resembles the words challenge or challenges. PRE/n is a proximity operator used exclusively in Scopus. (new PRE/2 nurse) means that the word "new" precedes the second word "nurse" by a number of words less than or equal to two words (www.help.scopus.com). The initial search parameters were set to all subject areas, search in titles, abstracts and keywords for articles or reviews published between January 2010 and December 2013. The search was further limited to Nursing, as a subject area, and to publications in English Language in the United States of America (USA), Australia, United Kingdom (UK), New Zealand, Canada, United Arab Emirates (UAE) and Lebanon. The Search returned 77 articles.

In CINAHL, the following Boolean phrase was used: ("novice nurse*" OR "novice registered nurse*" OR "new* graduat* nurse*" OR "new* licensed nurse*" OR "new* registered nurse*" OR "graduat* nurse*" OR "graduat* registered nurse*") AND (transition) AND (challenge* OR program*). The default search field was applied which included a search in the title, abstract and subject headings. The search was limited to research article publications in English Language, included abstract, full text and references, studies on Humans, published between Jan 2010 and December 2013 in the Middle-east, Africa, USA, Australia and New Zealand, UK and Ireland, and Canada. The search returned 13 articles.

In PubMed, the following Boolean phrase was used in the initial search: ("novice nurse" OR "new graduate nurse" OR "newly licensed nurse" OR "newly licensed registered nurse" OR "new registered nurse" OR "graduate nurse" OR "graduate registered nurse") AND (transition) AND (program OR challenge). The (*)

wildcard and the proximity operators were not applicable for use in this database. The search parameters were set for search in titles or abstracts, in studies on Human species, written in English Language, included abstracts and full text publications, and published between January 2010 and December 2013. The search rendered 23 articles.

The search outcome in the three databases rendered a total of 113 citations. All citations were uploaded to Refworks and duplicates were removed. The final result of citations for potential review was 84 articles (Figure 1).

3. Data Evaluation

The data evaluation process comprised the identification of the inclusion/ exclusion criteria (Table One). The inclusion/ exclusion criteria were formulated after reading through the titles, abstracts and the text of many articles captured during the data collection stage.

After finalizing the inclusion/ exclusion criteria, Refworks was used to review the full citations of the 84 articles. The articles that obviously met the exclusion criteria and did not meet the inclusion criteria were excluded. As a result, the list of articles went down to 55 articles which were downloaded and prepared for potential review.

The next step entailed the development of a tabulated form using Microsoft excel. Pertinent data retained from the full text articles were documented in the tabulated form. The data retained were related to research design, sample (type, size, gender, occupation, age), instrument, data analysis (statistical or other), country, variables/ factors, hypothesis/ objectives, results, and limitations. During this data evaluation step, articles which met any of the exclusion criteria were immediately excluded without further review of text information.

Table One	
Inclusion Criteria	**Exclusion Criteria**
1. Mainly address transition challenges among new graduate registered nurses 2. New graduate registered nurses with a professional practice experience less than or equal to 18 months. 3. Adult nursing practice 4. Acute care hospital settings 5. Studies from USA and from countries of which their first Language is Arabic Language. 6. Primary research	1. Not addressing transition challenges among new graduate nurses 2. New graduate nurses with more than 18 months of professional practice experience. 3. Non-adult nursing practice 4. Non-acute care hospital setting 5. In countries other than those specified in the inclusion criteria 6. Addressing advanced nursing practice (Nurse practitioners, clinical educators..) 7. Addressing transition of nurses from MSN (Master in Nursing) program. 8. Addressing transition of experienced registered nurses 9. Addressing transition of nurses from one country to another 10. Addressing transition into academic nursing education 11. PARISH nursing. 12. Registered/ Licensed midwives 13. Secondary research

As a result of this more detailed review with documentation of relevant information, the list went further down to 16 articles. Many articles were excluded due to one of the following reasons: 1) From excluded countries 2) Address student nurses, 2) have more than 18 months of professional practice experience, 3) Address advanced nurse practitioners 4) Address other specialty nursing like midwifery or pediatrics. The last step in the data evaluation process comprised a search for relevant articles in the bibliographic lists of the 16 articles. The final list rendered was 17 articles (Figure 1).

Figure One

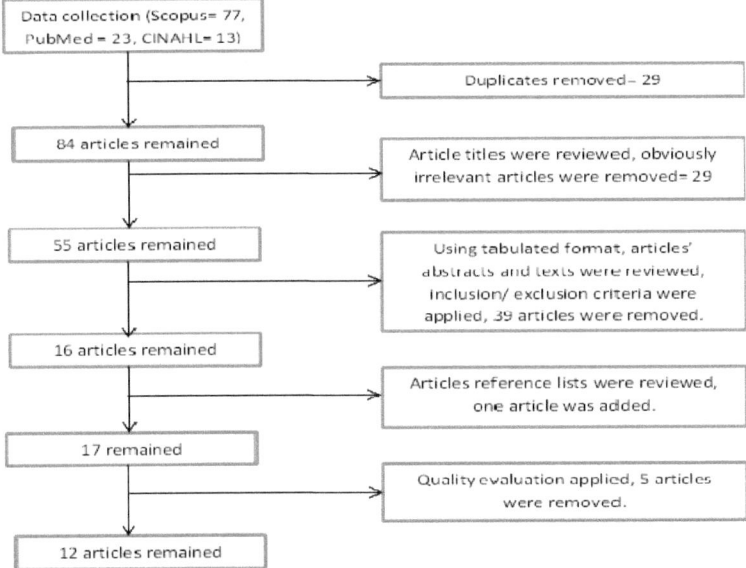

4. Data Analysis

The fourth stage in cooper's (1989) stages of integrative review implicates a description of the author's approach in conducting data analysis and interpretation. The analysis comprises an evaluation of the quality of articles obtained so that low quality articles are further excluded from the review.

A quality evaluation checklist was adapted from the quality evaluation index initially developed by Beck (2001) (Appendix A), modified by Park and Jones (2010) and adapted afterwards by Rush, Adamack, Gordon, Lilly and Janke (2013) (Appendix B). Three evaluation criteria which were most applicable to this review were adopted with minor modifications: a) research design (1= descriptive or qualitative, 2= longitudinal), b) sample size (1= less than 50, 2= 51-100, 3= 101-150, 4= 151-200, 5= more than 200), and c) instrument reliability and validity (0= reliability and validity are not reported, 1= reliability or validity for previous studies was reported,

13

2= reported the reliability or validity of the current study, 3= reported reliability and validity of the current study). The maximum score that can be reached in any article is 10 points which is the summation of the highest scores of the three criteria.

The articles which attained a score of five or higher were considered "high quality articles" and were included in the final analysis while the ones which scored four or below were considered low quality articles. Interestingly, all the three articles, addressing the population of interest in the Arabic speaking countries, attained a low quality score. However, these three articles are very important to include in this review because they are the only available publications addressing our main subject in the Arabic speaking countries. Hence, only five articles with low quality score were excluded and the remaining articles for review were reduced to 12 articles. The scores of the 17 articles are illustrated in Table Two.

Table Two

(Author, year)	a	b	c	Total (10)
(Ballard, Mead, Richardson, & Lotz, 2012)	1	1	0	2
(Bratt & Felzer, 2011)	2	5	2	9
(Clark & Springer, 2012)	1	1	2	4
(Dyess & Parker, 2012)	2	3	2	7
(Fielden, 2012)	1	1	2	4
(Goode, Lynn, McElroy, Bednash, & Murray, 2013)	2	5	3	10
(Holland & Moddeman, 2012)	2	1	2	5
(Kantar, 2012)	1	1	1	3
(Kowalski & Cross, 2010)	2	1	3	6
(Kramer, Brewer, & Maguire, 2013)	2	5	3	10
(Kramer, Maguire, Brewer, & Schmalenberg, 2013)	1	5	2	8
(Kramer et al., 2012)	1	5	2	8
(Maxwell, 2011)	2	1	3	6
(Moore & Cagle, 2012)	1	1	2	4
(Nematollahi & Isaac, 2012)	1	1	0	2
(Patterson, Bayley, Burnell, & Rhoads, 2010)	2	1	1	4
(Washington, 2012)	2	1	2	4

CHAPTER III

FINDINGS

A. **Methodological Implications**

The fifth stage in cooper's (1989) integrative research process entails presentation of the results. The methodological strategy followed herein provided important findings in regard to the availability of published literature addressing transition challenges of new graduate nurses. It is safe to conclude that this subject is well addressed internationally, specifically in USA, Australia, UK and Canada while, as echoed in Kantar (2012), limited research has been conducted in the Arabic speaking countries. The quality of such publications varies from one article to another. In USA, in the past three years, many research studies had large sample sizes representing regional or nation-wide populations. The research designs were qualitative, quantitative descriptive, longitudinal pre and post, and repeated measures designs. However, consistent with the research findings reported by Bratt & Felzer (2011), the literature lacked quasi-experimental or experimental designs which indicated inconclusive evidence and posed a gap in research for future consideration.

B. **Qualitative Findings**

1. *Themes Identified in the Arabic Speaking Countries*

Table Three illustrates the qualitative and quantitative findings of the selected research publications in this review. In Lebanon and the Kingdom of Saudi Arabia (KSA), both Fielden (2012) and Kantar (2012) report that NGNs focus on performing the tasks, procedures and techniques while delivering patient care rather than assuming a holistic patient care approach. Kantar (2012) particularly refers to this challenge as an "emphasis on implementing care and skill acquisition" while Fielden

15

(2012) refers to it as a "task focus rather than patient focus." The second transition challenge that NGNs experience is the limited critical thinking ability and the difficulty in organizing patient care (Fielden, 2012). This is supported by Kantar (2012) who further explains that the NGNs show mainly a limited ability to relate patient care to patient data. NGNs demonstrate a difficulty in anticipating patient changes and they depend on other professionals including their preceptors (third challenge) to identify patient changes, understand those changes and make the appropriate clinical decisions (Fielden, 2012; Kantar, 2012). However, the lack of support experienced by NGNs, the fourth challenge reported by Nematollahi & Isaac (2012) in the United Arab Emirates (UAE), can lead to NGN resignation. The fifth NGNs' transition challenge represents the difficulty in "understanding the complexities of people, health and nursing itself (Fielden, 2012). This is supported by Kantar (2012) who reports a "deficit in data collection" among NGN's. Other challenges reported in Lebanon and KSA include NGNs' difficulties in communicating effectively (Fielden, 2012, Kantar 2012), "adoption of a detached observer role" and dissatisfaction with their professional role (Fielden, 2012), "lack of self-evaluation prompt", "dependence on informal feedback" and dependence on knowledge gained from the nursing school curricula (Kantar, 2012).

2. The Arabic Speaking Countries Compared to USA

In USA, the quantitative findings reported by Kramer, Brewer & Maguire (2013) in relation to the role transition challenges of NGNs have been supported in a qualitative study by the same primary investigator Kramer et al., (2012). The sample size and type of both studies is fairly a nation-wide representative sample of the NGNs' population in the United States. Both studies supplement each other by providing strong evidence in concluding seven critical challenges that face NGNs in the United States. The seven challenges are summarized in Table Three in the more recent publication by the primary investigator Kramer et al., (2012).

A close look at the results shows a wide range of similarities in the transition challenges that NGNs encounter in both areas of the world. Delegation is one challenge common in Lebanon, KSA and USA. In USA, the NGN's challenge in delegating a task/ responsibility while preserving the accountability for it is exemplified in KSA and Lebanon in the NGNs difficulty in delivering holistic patient. Prioritization, another challenge identified among NGNs in USA, is exemplified in KSA where NGNs were noted to have difficulties in organizing patient care and demonstrating effective critical thinking abilities; whereas, in Lebanon, NGNs had difficulty in relating patient data to patient care which, indirectly, reflects difficulty in prioritizing patient care.

The third challenge, identified in Kramer, Brewer & Maguire (2013) and Kramer et al (2012) in USA, is the difficulty in the management of patient care delivery. This challenge is exemplified in KSA and Lebanon in many aspects not limited to NGNs dependence on curriculum knowledge, difficulty relating patient data to patient care, difficulty in anticipating patient care, showing deficits in data collection (Kantar 2012), difficulty in critically thinking and organizing patient care (Fielden, 2012).

Autonomous-decision making, the fourth challenge, is well exemplified in USA, Lebanon and KSA. NGNs depend on preceptors and other professionals in making clinical decisions. They frequently seek guidance and assistance in identifying, understanding and acting on patient changes. The fifth challenge "Utilizing feedback to restore self-confidence identified in Kramer, Brewer & Maguire (2013) and Kramer et al (2012) is also partially applicable to KSA where NGNs echo a dis-satisfaction with their professional role (Fielden, 2012) and to Lebanon where NGNs lack the self-evaluation initiative and depend on informal feedback about their performance (Kantar, 2012). In UAE, Nematollahi & Isaac

(2012) reported that the primary reason behind NGNs resignation was the lack of support of the nursing team. The lack of support exemplifies a the Bureaucratic system identified as a high concern at four months of hire for NGNs in Karmer, Brewere & Maguire (2013), and exemplifies the "reality generated stress" categorized under "Utilizing feedback to restore confidence" in Kramer et al (2012).

The remaining two challenges "Collaboration with other disciplines" and "Constructive conflict resolution" reported in USA are not clearly exemplified in the two studies conducted in KSA and Lebanon. However, both studies in USA and Lebanon identified a lack in effective communication among NGNs. Effective communication constitutes a challenge integrated in the "collaboration" and "conflict resolution" challenges. Effective communication is the mechanism utilized to establish a collaborative work environment and to resolve conflicts constructively.

Table Three			
Author/ Country	Design	Sample	Findings
(Bratt & Felzer, 2011)/ USA	Quant., repeated measures design	428 NGNs	• Significant improvement over time on clinical decision making, job satisfaction, organizational commitment and quality of nursing performance. • Significant reduction over time on job stress.
(Dyess & Parker, 2012)/ USA	Quant. Longitud.	109 NGNs	• Significant improvement over time on four subscales of skill acquisition: planning and evaluation, member of the discipline, leading care and patient care. • No significant improvement on communication subscale.
(Goode et al., 2013)/ USA	Quant., Repeated measures design	1016 NGNs	• Significant improvement over time on resident's perceptions of their overall confidence and competence, organizing and prioritizing, communication, and leadership. • Professional satisfaction scores decreased significantly at 6 months and remained close to the 6 month level at completion of program.
(Holland & Moddeman, 2012)/ USA	Quant., Repeated measures design	24 NGNs	• Increased mean total scores for the Casey-Fink instrument over time indicated improved confidence levels. • Significant improvement over time on the organizing-prioritizing and communication-leadership subscales. • Feeling supported was highest at the beginning of their residency program with slightly decrease over time.

Author/ Country	Design	Sample	Findings
Table Three			
			• Mean scores of professional satisfaction decreased slightly over time.
(Kowalski & Cross, 2010)/ USA	Quant., Pre and Post	Pre: below 50 NGNs, post below 20 NGNs	• Significant improvement in critical thinking and clinical competency over time. • NGNs feelings of being threatened or challenged decreased over time. • Significant decrease was noted on feelings of being threatened. • Non-significant decrease in overall anxiety levels. • Casey-fink instrument results: o Significant improvement on communication-leadership subscale o Non-significant improvement on the support, professional satisfaction and safety subscales.
(Kramer, Brewer, & Maguire, 2013)/ USA	Quant., repeated measure, comparative.	468 NGNs	• High concern at 4 and 8 months: o Get work done o Lack of self-confidence o Harm patient o Delegation o Prioritization o Working with physicians o Not enough feedback o Too much responsibility o Float to other units • No or some Concern at 4 months, High at 8 months: o Patients do not receive needed care o Friction, disagreement, Conflict • High concern at 4 months, some or no concern at 8 months: o Not like taught in school o Role expectation exceed preparation o Physical labor- mental fatigue o Work-life imbalance o Bureaucratic system • Significant differences in degree of Environmental Reality Shock experienced by new graduates at 4, 8, and 12 months post hire. • NGNs working on units with confirmed Very Healthy Work Environments experience less Environmental Reality Shock than do their peers working on other units.
(Kramer et	Mixed,	907	• Results focus on characteristics of nurse residency

19

Table Three			
Author/ Country	**Design**	**Sample**	**Findings**
al., 2013)/ USA	Qual., Quant., descript.	(same sample for Kramer et al., 2012)	programs which do not answer any of the research questions of this review.

(Kramer et al., 2012)/ USA	Mixed method, primarily qual.	907 (330 NGNs, 401 Preceptors, 138 managers and 38 educators), nationally representative sample	NGN critical challenges in the management of professional role responsibilities:
			• Delegation
			  o Accountability/ Responsibility issue
			• Prioritization
			  o NGNs prioritize patients rather than tasks and activities
			  o NGNs do not understand the unit priority system.
			• Managing patient care delivery
			  o Getting the work done, coping with high information intake and output, managing the therapeutic environments for multiple patients and fear of harming patients.
			  o Difficulty understanding the nursing care delivery system on the unit.
			• Autonomous-decision making
			• Collaboration with other disciplines
			  o NGN- physician collaboration is affected by the NGN's lack of competency and self-confidence in addition to the lack of structure and opportunity for collaboration.
			• Constructive conflict resolution
			  o Delegation is the primary source of NGN-specific conflict.
			• Utilizing feedback to restore self-confidence.
			  o Expectation-reality generated stress.
			  o Unclear statement of goals and expected role performance
			  o Premature signaling of readiness to perform when competence is not established.

(Maxwell, 2011)/ USA	Quant., descript., longitud.	37 NGNs	• Organizing- prioritizing, communication- leadership, and support scores on the Casey-fink instrument increased over time. • Significant reduction in stress scores was noted overtime. • Professional satisfaction decreased over time although the

20

Table Three			
Author/ Country	**Design**	**Sample**	**Findings**
			scores were high over the duration of the program.
(Fielden, 2012) / KSA	Qual.	18 NGNs	Perception of experience: • "Dissatisfaction with role and high standard of care expected of NGNs." Knowledge: • "Incomplete understanding of the complexities of people, health and nursing itself." Critical thinking: • "Limited ability to think in either a reflective or an anticipatory way." Communication: • Difficulties in communication Role: • "Adoption of a detached observer role." Focus: "Task focus rather than patient focus."
(Kantar, 2012) / Lebanon	Qual., multiple case study	21 NGNs	Noticing: • "Dependence on knowledge from the curriculum" • "Deficits in data collection" • "Reliance on data identified by others" Interpreting: • "Difficulty relating care orders to changes" • "Less attentive to changes in clinical status" • "Dependence on others to understand changes" Responding: • "Ineffective communication" • "Emphasis on implementing care and skill acquisition" • "Seek guidance from experienced others" • "Emphasis on procedures and techniques" Reflecting: • "Lack self-evaluation prompt" • "Dependence on informal feedback"
(Nematollahi & Isaac, 2012) / UAE	Qual.	5 NGNs	The main reason for resignation: • Lack of support from nursing administration, in-charge nurses and preceptors.

C. Quantitative Findings

The quantitative findings provide further support for the existence of the role transition challenges reflected in the themes discussed earlier. However, the findings are only specific to USA and cannot be compared to the Arabic speaking countries because of the Lack of such research in the latter countries.

1. *Overall confidence and competence*

Using the Casey-Fink Graduate Nurse Experience Survey (2004), NGNs' perceptions of their overall confidence and competence indicated a significant improvement over time during the implementation of a residency program. Furthermore, the results of the Casey-Fink survey indicated a significantly more improvement in Magnet "A" hospitals in comparison to non-magnet hospitals (Goode, Lynn, McElroy, Bednash, & Murray, 2013). This is consistent with the findings reported in Holland & Moddeman, (2012) which indicated an improvement in the overall perceptions of confidence of NGNs participating in a residency program.

2. *Prioritization-organization skills*

NGN's perceptions of their overall prioritization-organization skills have improved significantly over time during the nurse residency program. Additionally, a significantly more improvement was noted in Magnet "A" hospitals when compared to non-magnet hospitals (Goode, Lynn, McElroy, Bednash, & Murray, 2013). This finding is consistent findings reported in Holland & Moddeman (2012) and Maxwell (2011). The Casey-Fink Graduate Nurse Experience Survey (2004) was used in the three studies.

3. *Communication-leadership skills*

Again, Using the Casey-Fink Graduate Nurse Experience surveys (2004, 2002) and over the period of nurse residency program implementation, Significant improvement on NGNs' perceptions of their overall communication-leadership skills was noted. Also, NGNs' in Magnet "A" hospitals showed a significantly more improvement when compared to non-magnet hospitals (Goode, Lynn, McElroy, Bednash, & Murray, 2013). This finding is consistent with the findings reported in all of the selected studies using the Casey-Fink survey particularly for the significant improvement noted on the communication-leadership skills over the period of the residency program (Holland & Moddeman, 2012; Kowalski & Cross, 2010; Maxwell, 2011). However, using the Nurse Evaluation Competency Assessment tool (NECA) developed by Shwirian (1978) and revised by Turansky (2003), a non-significant improvement on communication subscale was noted (Dyess & Parker, 2012).

4. Clinical competency

A variety of tools were used to evaluate the clinical competency of NGNs during their participation in residency programs. Using the clinical decision making scale (Jenkins, 1985) and the Modified 6-D scale of nursing performance developed by (Schwirian, 1978) and revised by (Marshalleck 1997), Bratt & Felzer (2011) reported a significant improvement in clinical decision making and quality of nursing performance respectively. On the other hand, Kowalski & Cross (2010) reported a significant improvement in critical thinking and clinical competency but a non-significant improvement in safety practices. The safety practices were evaluated using the older version of the Casey-Fink Graduate Nurse Experience Survey (2002) whereas critical thinking and clinical competency were evaluated using the preceptor evaluation of resident- an instrument developed and validated by a panel of expert nurse clinicians in the hospital.

5. Professional satisfaction

NGNs' professional satisfaction scores showed little variation in results from one study to another. Using the Casey-Fink instrument, in two studies out of four

23

studies, the authors reported a decrease in professional satisfaction scores over time (Holland & Moddeman, 2012; Maxwell, 2011). In the third study, the scores decreased significantly by the end of the first 6 month period of the residency program and stayed almost at the same level at the end of the program (Goode, Lynn, McElroy, Bednash, & Murray, 2013). However, Kowalski & Cross (2010) reported a non- significant increase in professional satisfaction over time. This last finding, which is opposite to the findings in the other three studies, may be attributed to the low response rate (n=14) at the end of the program compared to a much higher response rate at the beginning of the program (n=37).

6. Perceived support

Using Casey-Fink instrument, Holland & Moddeman (2012) reported that "Feeling supported" decreased slightly over time. Goode et al., (2013) reported significant decrease over the first 6 months period followed by an increase over the next 6 months period. Both Kowalski & Cross (2012) and Maxwell (2011) reported that support scores increased over time.

7. Job stress

Both Maxwell (2011) and Bratt & Felzer (2011) reported a reduction in stress levels among NGNs over the duration of the residency programs. Bratt & Felzer (2011) particularly reported a significant reduction over time. Maxwell (2011) utilized the Casey-Fink instrument (2004) while Bratt & Felzer (2011) utilized the Job Stress Scale (Hinshaw and Atwood, 1985).

8. Summary of quantitative findings

All of the selected studies for this review indicated that the NGNs' overall confidence and competence, organization- prioritization skills, communication-leadership skills and clinical competency had significantly improved over the period of the Nurse Residency programs (NRPs). The results on the NGNs' perceptions of support as well as the professional satisfaction had varied from one study to another.

D. Instruments

In the all of the 8 quantitative studies selected for this review, a total of 15 instruments were used to measure NGNs' role transition issues. The Casey-Fink Graduate Nurse Experience Survey was used in four studies whereas each of the remaining instruments was only used in one study only. Goode, Lynn, McElroy, Bednash, & Murray (2013) utilized the Casey-Fink instrument, had a repeated measures design, and had the largest sample size (n=1016) of all the studies. This study used the Casey-Fink instrument as the only measurement tool to measure the transition challenges "Support", "Organizing-Prioritizing", "Communication-leadership", "Stress" and "Professional Satisfaction". The overall reliability coefficient was equal to 0.89 in this study and ranged from 0.73 to 0.82 for its subscales. The other instrument used in this study was the Graduate Nurse Residency Program Evaluation (GNRPE) which is a tool designed to evaluate NGNs' satisfaction about the residency program. Similarly in Maxwell (2011) (sample size= 37), and Holland & Moddeman (2012) (sample size= 24), the only tool used to measure transition challenges was the Casey-Fink instrument. The reliability coefficient for the Casey-Fink instrument in Maxwell (2011) was equal to 0.89 whereas it was not reported in Holland & Moddeeman (2012). In Kowalski & Cross (2012) (sample size below 50, reliability estimate 0.71-0.9), the Casey-Fink instrument was used in addition to other tools each of which measures one specific challenge ("Stress", "Anxiety" and "clinical competence").

Table Four			
Author/ Country	Instrument	Reliability	Validity
(Bratt & Felzer, 2011)/ USA	Clinical decision making in Nursing Scale.	Alpha 0.82-0.83. Total alpha= 0.95, subscale= 0.71-0.90.	By original authors
	Modified 6-D scale of Nursing performance.	Total alpha= 0.9, subscale= 0.77-0.90.	
	The nurse job satisfaction scale.	total alpha= 0.87, subscale= 0.64=0.81.	
	Job stress scale. Organizational commitment questionnaire	Total alpha= 0.9-0.91	
(Dyess & Parker, 2012)/ USA	NECA	Overall alpha 0.94. For subscales: Pre 0.77-0.88, post 0.81-0.89.	By previous study
(Goode et al., 2013)/ USA	Casey-fink (2004)	Overall alpha= 0.89. Factors: Support= 0.82, organizing and prioritizing (0.76), stress (0.73), professional satisfaction (0.76, Communication / leadership (0.74).	Face validity.
(Holland & Moddeman, 2012)/ USA	Casey-fink (2004)	Reliability was examined with statistical analysis.	Not reported.
(Kowalski & Cross, 2010)/ USA	Preceptor evaluation of resident,	Reliability was discussed,	Discussed validity of all instruments.
	Casey-fink (2002),	Estimates 0.71-0.9.	
	Pagana's clinical stress questionnaire,	Reliability 0.84 and 0.85.	
	State-Trait anxiety inventory,	Reliability consistently above 0.9.	
(Kramer, Brewer, & Maguire, 2013)/ USA	ERS, EOMII, APPE, PPPE, QC	All were developed by authors. Reliability for all tools was determined. ERS is built depending on three sources, one of which is the Casey-fink 2004.	Validity was reported.
(Kramer et al., 2013)/ USA	RPQ	Developed by authors. No report on reliability.	Validated.
(Kramer et al.,	Interviews	Interview questions developed by	Validated.

26

Table Four			
Author/ Country	**Instrument**	**Reliability**	**Validity**
2012)/ USA		authors.	
(Maxwell, 2011)/ USA	Casey-fink (2004)	Reliability= 0.89	Validated
(Fielden, 2012) / KSA	Individual and group interviews, semi-structured questions	N/A	Validated.
(Kantar, 2012) / Lebanon	Individual interviews	N/A	Validated.
(Nematollahi & Isaac, 2012) / UAE	Phone interviews, individual	N/A	Not mentioned.

Table Four footnotes:

Casey-Fink: Casey-Fink Graduate Nurse Experience Survey (Casey, Fink, Krugman, & Propst, 2004)

Casey-Fink (2002): Casey-Fink Graduate Nurse Experience Survey (Casey, Fink, Krugman, & Propst, 2004)

NECA: Nursing Evaluation Competency Assessment tool (Schwirian 1978; J. Turansky, 2003)

Clinical decision making in nursing scale (Jenkins, 1985)

Modified 6-D scale of nursing performance (Schwirian, 1978), revised by (Marshalleck 1997).

The nurse job satisfaction scale (Hinshaw and Atwood, 1985).

Job stress scale (Hinshaw and Atwood, 1985).

Organizational commitment questionnaire (Mowday, Steers, and Porter, 1979).

Preceptor evaluation of resident (Kowalski & Cross, 2010).

Pagana's Clinical stress questionnaire (Pagana, K., 1989).

Spielberger's State-Trait anxiety inventory (Spielberger, C., 1983).

EOMII: Essentials of Magnetism II (Schmalenberg & Kramer, 2008).

ERS: Environmental Realty Shock (Kramer, Brewer, & Maguire, 2011).

APPE: Anticipated professional practice Environment (Kramer, Brewer, & Maguire, 2011).

PPPE: Perceived professional practice environment (Kramer, Brewer, & Maguire, 2011).

QC: Quality of patient care rating scale. This is a global 10-point, single-item indicator (Kramer, Brewer, & Maguire, 2011).

RPQ: Residency program Questionnaire (Kramer, Maguire, Halfer, Brewer, & Schmalenberg, 2013).

This tool is used in individual and group interviews to collect quantitative data.

Dyess & Parker (2012) (sample size= 109) utilized the NECA instrument which measures the Acquisition of clinical psychosocial and technical skills and the student Leadership Practice Inventory (SLPI). The NECA measures five dimensions of practice which are: planning and evaluation, patient care, communication, member of the discipline and leading care. The overall reliability coefficient for the NECA in this study was reported 0.94. Bratt & Felzer (2011) utilized several instruments each of which measuring a specific challenge dimension. In Kramer, Brewer & Maguire (2013), a large sample study (n= 468), the Environmental Reality Shock (ERS) instrument was utilized (Appendix C). The authors of this article utilized three sources to develop this ERS. One of these sources was the Casey-Fink instrument. Table Four below provides an overview of the instruments used.

To conclude the results for the Instruments, The Casey-Fink graduate Nurse Experience Survey (2004) was most frequently used by researchers. It was also used on the largest sample size of all the studies selected for this review. It covers the main themes reported as challenges for the NGNs and it is a reliable and valid instrument for measuring NGNs' transition challenges. The second important instrument is the ERS which is a comprehensive tool measuring all aspects of the Environment that the NGNs face. The other instruments are also good instruments but were not used as frequently and were limited to measure specific themes only.

CHAPTER IV

DISCUSSION

The little variation in the findings between Lebanon, KSA and USA can be attributed to the lack of recent research addressing this subject in the Arabic speaking countries. Only three publications were found in the Arabic speaking countries addressing this subject. One of the three studies addressing NGNs in UAE was only a report of the author's recommendations based on literature review rather than an empirical research study. The two other research publications in Lebanon and KSA followed qualitative designs which make them comparable only to other qualitative designs in USA. The themes identified in Lebanon, KSA and USA demonstrated a variation in the "titles" or "subject headings" synthesized by the respective authors; however, the content under all of the themes are similar in the three countries except that the studies in USA had a more comprehensive description of challenges and showed stronger evidence illustrated by the strong research designs and the sample types and sizes. This indicates that more research in this field should be carried out in the Arabic speaking countries in order to make a more valid and comprehensive comparison.

The variation in the qualitative findings can also be attributed to the different theories/models that the respective authors followed in conducting their studies and in synthesizing the themes identified. In Lebanon, Kantar (2012) used Tanner's (2006) model of clinical judgment in nursing as a guiding framework. The author synthesized the narrative data into themes along the "Noticing", "interpreting", "responding" and "reflection" stages of clinical judgment in Tanner's (2006) model. In KSA, both Fielden (2012) and Nematollahi & Isaac (2012) referred to Benner's (2001) model "From Novice to Expert" as a guiding framework in their respective studies. In USA, many theories were also used as guiding frameworks such the Systems Research Organizing Model (SROM) (Brewer, Verran, & Stichler, 2008) and the "knowing" , "becoming" and "affirming" stages of new nursing graduate professional role transition (Duchscher, 2008).

Only one large scale, high quality, qualitative study was found in USA literature in the past three years. The rest of the studies retrieved in USA were basically quantitative studies that provided strong evidence in support of the existence of NGNs' role transition challenges and demonstrated the efficacy of residency programs. There are much more abundant qualitative and quantitative studies addressing NGNs' transition issues before year 2010. This subject was initially addressed in 1974 when the author (Kramer, M., 1974) related nursing staff attrition to the reality shock they experience during transition into practice. In the past three years, research studies were more focused into studying the efficacy of residency programs through using quantitative designs. This indicates that the role transition challenges are realized now as a reality experienced in USA and other countries like Lebanon and KSA. The surplus of research publications, which has been published since 1974, supports the existence of role transition challenges and its negative effects on NGNs' retention (Clark & Springer, 2012; Fielden, 2012; Holland & Moddeman, 2012; Kramer, Maguire, Halfer, Brewer, & Schmalenberg, 2013; Rush, Adamack, Gordon, Lilly, & Janke, 2013).

In this research review, 15 different instruments were used to study role transition issues and residency program efficacy. The instruments used and the results reported out of it support the existence of the themes identified through 38 years of research in the field (since 1974). The instruments also provided valid and reliable evidence supporting the efficacy of residency programs in supporting NGNs' in their transition into professional practice (Bratt & Felzer, 2011; Dyess & Parker, 2012; Fielden, 2012; Goode, Lynn, McElroy, Bednash, & Murray, 2013; Kowalski &

Cross, 2010; Kramer et al., 2012; Kramer, Maguire, Brewer, & Schmalenberg, 2013; Maxwell, 2011). However, the instruments varied in their abilities to provide a comprehensive quantitative measurement of transition challenges. The two instruments, "Casey-Fink" and "ERS" had most of the transition themes represented in addition to being utilized in large scale, strongly designed studies that were accomplished by well experienced authors in the field.

CHAPTER V

LIMITATIONS

This study focused particularly on identifying the challenges in role transition that are shared between the Arabic speaking countries and USA. The study also provided an insight into the most appropriate instruments used to quantify those challenges. However, this study did not assess for the quality, design, and content of the nurse residency programs that had yielded positive results in smoothing role transition challenges and improving retention of NGNs. This limitation represents a valid research question that should be considered in future research studies. The second limitation is demonstrated in the methodology of this study where only one author executed the data collection, the data evaluation and the data analysis stages. The data collection, application of inclusion/ exclusion criteria and quality evaluation should be conducted by more than one author in order to ensure objectivity in the selection of articles for review.

CHAPTER VI

CONCLUSION

The major role transition challenges that are identified in USA, Lebanon and KSA are the ones represented in the Casey-Fink graduate Nurse Experience Survey (2004) which measures the overall confidence and competence of NGNs and is divided into five subscales: "Support" "Organizing-Prioritizing", "communication-Leadership", "Professional satisfaction" and "Stress". The "clinical competence" is a well identified challenge exemplified in studies not using the Casey-Fink instrument. However, this challenge is integrated in the overall competence and confidence of the Casey-Fink instrument.

The findings support the need to design residency programs that extend over a period of more than 6 months in order to ensure successful role transition of NGNs into workforce. The findings also indicate the importance of the use of the Casey-Fink instrument (2004) in studying NGNs' progress against the challenges that they face during their transition to practice and also in evaluating the efficacy and effectiveness of the transition programs. Yet, the instrument should be assessed for reliability and validity in the Arabic speaking countries before use in those countries. The instrument is only available for use by contacting its authors (Casey, Fink, Krugman, & Propst, 2004).

This review of the literature strongly indicates the need for more studies to learn about the NGNs' challenges and the strategies used by healthcare leaders to address this issue in the Arabic speaking countries. It is of particular concern that there are no quantitative studies that address NGNs' role transition issues in the Arabic speaking countries.

APPENDICES

APPENDIX A: Beck (2001) Quality Evaluation Index

Score	0	1	2	3	4
Author Expertise	N/A	Bachelor or MSN degree	PhD, MD or other Doctoral degree	Doctoral degree plus published multiple on postpartum depression (PPD) as the first author	N/A
Funding	Did not receive funding	Received funding	N/A	N/A	N/A
Sampling		Convenience	matched	Random	N/A
Sample Size	N/A	1-50	51-100	More than 100	N/A
PPD Instrument	No mention of reliability or validity	Mention of only previous reliability and/ or validity	Addressed reliability or validity in current study	Addressed reliability and validity of current study	Combination of 1 & 3.
Predictor instrument	No mention of reliability or validity	Mention of only previous reliability and/ or validity	Addressed reliability or validity in current study	Addressed reliability and validity of current study	Combination of 1 & 3.
Depression measurement	N/A	Self-report	Unstructured interview	Diagnosis based on specified criteria	N/A
PPD type	N/A	Only measured depressive symptomatology	Diagnosis of PPD was made	N/A	N/A
Research Design	N/A	Descriptive	Correlational	Quasi-Experimental	Experimental
Time dimensional design	N/A	Cross Sectional	Longitudinal	N/A	N/A
Data Analysis	N/A	Descriptive Statistics	Non-parametric statistics	Bivariate statistics	Multi-variate statistics

APPENDIX B: Rush, Adamack, Gordon, Lilly, and Janke (2013) Quality Evaluation

Score	1	2	3
Research Design	Descriptive and Qualitative	Longitudinal	Quasi-Experimental
Sample Size	0-50	51-100	Greater than 100
Author Expertise	Less than 3 publications in transition program literature	More than 3 publications in transition program literature	N/A

APPENDIX C: Items in the Environmental Reality Shock Instrument

- Getting my work done on time.
- Harming patient due to inexperience.
- Prioritizing patient care.
- Things are not done the way I was taught in school.
- Role expectations exceed what I was prepared for.
- "Floating" to other units.
- Delegating work to nurse aides and technicians.
- "Weight" of too much responsibility.
- I find my work dull, routine, and monotonous.
- Not enough feedback—do not know how I am doing.
- There is a lot of friction, blaming, and fault finding.
- Patients do not receive the quantity or quality of care.
- Physical labor and resulting mental and physical fatigue.
- Competing life interests—work-life imbalance.
- Working with dying patients and their families.
- Unfair rules, policies, and treatment.
- Working within the system and the bureaucracy.
- Fitting in with the unit staff—I am still an outsider.
- Developing and building my self-confidence as a nurse.
- Working with physicians.
- Want to be independent but lack confidence.
- Inconsistent support from manager, preceptors, other.

BIBLIOGRAPHY

Ballard, J., Mead, C., Richardson, D., & Lotz, A. (2012). Impact of disease-specific orientation on new graduate nurse satisfaction and knowledge retention. *Journal of Neuroscience Nursing, 44*(3), 168-174.

Beck, C.T., (2001). Predictors of postpartum depression: an update. Nursing Research,
50(5), 275-285.

Benner P. (2001). From Novice to Expert: Excellence and Power in Clinical Nursing practice, Commemorative Edition. Prentice Hall, Upper Saddle River, NJ.

Bratt, M. M., & Felzer, H. M. (2011). Perceptions of professional practice and work environment of new graduates in a nurse residency program. *Journal of Continuing Education in Nursing, 42*(12), 559-568.

Brewer, B. B., Verran, J. A., & Stichler, J. L. (2008). The systems research organizing model: A conceptual perspective for facilities design. *Health Environments Research and Design Journal*, 1(4), 7-19.

Canadian Nurses Association, (2007). Tested solutions for eliminating Canada's registered nursing shortage.

Casey K., Fink R., Krugman M. & Propst J. (2004). The graduate nurse experience. *The Journal of Nursing Administration, 34*, 303–311.

Clark, C. M., & Springer, P. J. (2012). Nurse residents' first-hand accounts on transition to practice. *Nursing Outlook, 60*(4), e2-e8.

Cooper, H.M., (1989). The integrative research review: A systematic approach. Sage, Newbury Park.

Duchscher, J. E. B. (2008). A process of becoming: The stages of new nursing graduate professional role transition. *Journal of Continuing Education in Nursing*, 39, 441-450.

Dyess, S., & Sherman, R. (2011). Developing the leadership skills of new graduates to influence practice environments: A novice nurse leadership program. *Nursing Administration Quarterly, 35*(4), 313-322.

El-Jardali, F., Dimassi, H., Dumit, N., Jamal, D., Mouro, G., (2009a). A National Cross-sectional Study on Nurses' Intent to Leave and Job Satisfaction in Lebanon: Implications for Policy and Practice. *BMC Nursing* 8, 3.

El-Jardali, F., Dumit, N., Jamal, D., Mouro, G., (2008). Migration of Lebanese nurses: a questionnaire survey and secondary data analysis. *International Journal of Nursing Studies*, 45 (10), 1490–1500.

El-Jardali, F., Jamal, D., Abdallah, A., Kassak, K., (2007). Human resources for health planning and management in the Eastern Mediterranean region: facts, gaps and forward thinking for research and policy. *Human Resources for Health Journal* 5, 9.

El-Jardali, F., Longuenesse, E., Jamal, D., Kronfol, N., (2012). Health workforce in the Arab world: a public health challenge. In: Jabbour, S., Giacaman, R., Khawaja, M., Nuwayhid, I. (Eds.), *Public Health in the Arab World*. Cambridge University Press.

El-Jardali, F., Merhi, M., Dumit, N., Jamal, D., (2009b). Assessment of nurse retention challenges and practices in Lebanese hospitals: the perspective of nursing directors. *Journal of Nursing Management* 17, 453–462.

El-Jardali, F., Murray, S., Dimassi, H., Jamal, D., AbuAlRub, R., Al-Surimi, K., Clinton, M., Dumit, N., (2013). Intention to stay of nurses in current posts in difficult-to-staff areas of Yemen, Jordan, Lebanon and Qatar: A cross-sectional study. *International Journal of Nursing Studies*, http://dx.doi.org/10.1016/j.ijnurstu.2013.02.013.

Fielden, J. M. (2012). Managing the transition of saudi new graduate nurses into clinical practice in the kingdom of saudi arabia. *Journal of Nursing Management, 20*(1), 28-37.

Goode, C. J., Lynn, M. R., McElroy, D., Bednash, G. D., & Murray, B. (2013). Lessons learned from 10 years of research on a post-baccalaureate nurse residency program. *Journal of Nursing Administration, 43*(2), 73-79.

Hinshaw, A. S., & Atwood, J. R. (1985). *Anticipated turnover among nursing staff study: Final report.* National Institutes of Health. National Center of Nursing Research.

Holland, C., & Moddeman, G. R. (2012). Transforming the journey for newly licensed registered nurses. *Journal of Continuing Education in Nursing, 43*(7), 330-336.

Institute of Medicine. (2010). The future of nursing: leading change, advancing health.

Jenkins, H. M. (1985). A research tool for measuring perceptions of clinical decision making. *Journal of Professional Nursing, 1*(4), 221- 229.

Kantar, L. D. (2012). Clinical practice of new nurse graduates in lebanon: Challenges and perspectives through the eyes of preceptors. *Journal of Continuing Education in Nursing, 43*(11), 518-528.

Kovner, C. T., Brewer, C. S., Fairchild, S., Poornima, S., Kim, H., & Djukic, M. (2007). Newly licensed RNs, characteristics, work attitudes, and intentions to work. American Journal of Nursing, 107(9), 58Y70.

Kowalski, S., & Cross, C. L. (2010). Preliminary outcomes of a local residency programme for new graduate registered nurses. *Journal of Nursing Management, 18*(1), 96-104.

Kramer, M., (1974). Reality Shock: Why Nurses Leave Nursing. Mosby, Saint Louis.

Kramer, M., Brewer, B., & Maguire, P. (2013). Impact of healthy work environments on new graduate nurses' environmental reality shock. *Western Journal of Nursing Research*, 35(3), 348-383.

Kramer, M., Maguire, P., Halfer, D., Brewer, B., & Schmalenberg, C. (2013). Impact of residency programs on professional socialization of newly licensed registered nurses. *Western Journal of Nursing Research,* 35(4), 459-496.

Kramer, M., Maguire, P., Halfer, D., Budin, W. C., Hall, D. S., Goodloe, L., . . . Lemke, J. (2012). The organizational transformative power of nurse residency programs. *Nursing Administration Quarterly, 36*(2), 155-168.

Marshalleck, E. F. (1997). *The effect of education, job characteristics, and hospital unit structure on nurse performance and job satisfaction* (Unpublished doctoral dissertation). Stanford University, Palo Alto, CA.

Maxwell, K. L. (2011). The implementation of the UHC/AACN new graduate nurse residency program in a community hospital. *Nursing Clinics of North America, 46*(1), 27-33.

Moore, P., & Cagle, C. S. (2012). The lived experience of new nurses: Importance of the clinical preceptor. *Journal of Continuing Education in Nursing, 43*(12), 555-565.

Mowday, R. T., Steers, R. M., & Porter, L. W. (1979). The measurement of organizational commitment. *Journal of Vocational Behavior, 14,* 224-247.

Nematollahi, R., & Isaac, J. P. (2012). Bridging the theory practice gap: A review of graduate nurse program (GNP) in dubai, united arab emirates. *International Nursing Review, 59*(2), 194-199.

National Center for Health Workforce Analysis, (2002). Projected supply, demand, and shortages of registered nurses: 2000–2020.

Nursing Executive Center. (2005). Bridging the preparation-practice gap. Washington, DC: Author.

Pagana K. (1989). Psychometric evaluation of the clinical stress questionnaire (CSQ). *Journal of Nursing Education*, 28, 169–174.

Park, M., & Jones, C.B., (2010). A retention strategy for newly graduated nurses. Journal for Nurses in Staff Development, 26(4), 142-149.

Patterson, B., Bayley, E. W., Burnell, K., & Rhoads, J. (2010). Orientation to emergency nursing: Perceptions of new graduate nurses. *Journal of Emergency Nursing, 36*(3), 203-211.

Schwirian, P. M. (1978). Evaluating the performance of nurses: A multidimensional approach. *Nursing Research, 27*(6), 347-351.

Spielberger C. (1983). *State-Trait Anxiety Inventory (Form Y)*. Mind Garden Publishers, Redwood City, CA.

Tanner, C. A. (2006). Thinking like a nurse: A research-based model of clinical judgment in nursing. *Journal of Nursing Education*, 45(6), 204-211.

Turansky J. (2003) Assessment of nursing educational outcomes. Unpublished dissertation. University of Delaware.

Washington, G. T. (2012). Performance anxiety in new graduate nurses: Is it for real? *Dimensions of Critical Care Nursing*, 31(5), 295-300.

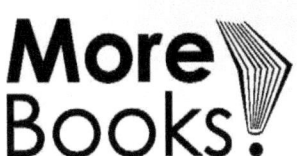
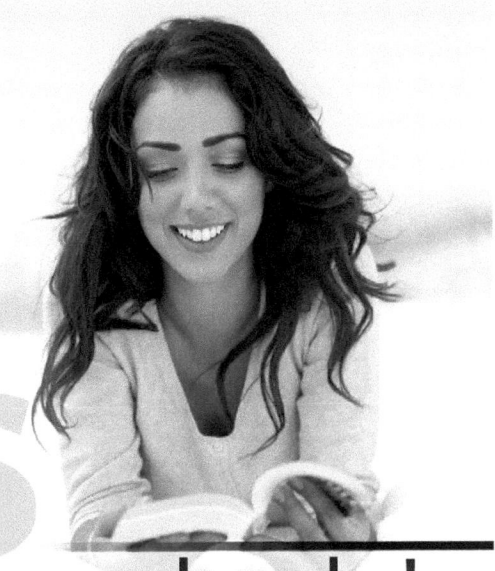
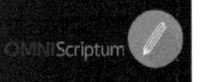

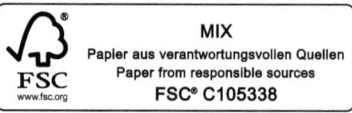
Printed by Books on Demand GmbH, Norderstedt / Germany